ATHLETE'S FOOT

I0421946

Approaches to Prevention, Treatment, and Relief from Athlete's Foot: An Exhaustive Handbook

CARL JUAN

Table of Contents

Introductory

Common fungal infections of the feet include athlete's foot, also called tinea pedis. The term "athlete's foot" refers to a fungal infection that is commonly seen on the feet of those who engage in strenuous physical activity and whose feet are constantly in close contact with communal surfaces like gym floors and locker room shower stalls. However, anyone can develop athlete's foot, not just athletes.

• Trichophyton is the most frequent fungus responsible for the illness. The feet are a perfect breeding ground for these fungi because of their warm, damp conditions. Itching, burning, redness, peeling, and cracking skin are common signs of athlete's foot, which is most common between the toes and on the soles of the feet. In some cases, blisters may occur, and the infection can spread to other parts of the foot or to the toenails.

• If you ignore athlete's foot, it can become painful and difficult to treat. It's also possible for it to be contagious, spreading from person to person via droplets or contaminated surfaces. Athlete's foot can be prevented or treated by always keeping feet clean and dry, by wearing shoes that allow air circulation, and by applying an over-the-counter antifungal cream or powder. A doctor may decide to administer stronger antifungal medicine for more severe cases.

CHAPTER ONE
Athletic Foot: The Fundamentals

Athlete's foot, also known as tinea pedis, is a fungal illness that typically manifests itself between the toes and on the soles of the feet. The fundamentals of athlete's foot are as follows:

1. Trichophyton, the most common form of fungus, is the root cause of athlete's foot. Fungi like your sweaty feet, especially communal areas like shower floors and locker rooms, where the air is warm and damp.

2. There is a wide variety of symptoms that can accompany athlete's foot.

• The discomfort of itching in the affected area is a common complaint.

Some patients report a burning feeling wherever the infection is present.

• **Redness:** The skin may get red, especially in the space between the toes.

The skin may begin to peel, and in more extreme situations, it may crack.

- Blisters: In some circumstances, the disorder may create fluid-filled blisters.

- **Odor:** Athlete's foot can lead to foul-smelling feet.

3. Transmission: Athlete's foot is contagious and can be passed on through intimate contact with an infected individual or contaminated surfaces. Good cleanliness and not sharing personal items like towels, socks, and shoes are essential for preventing the transmission of disease.

4. Athlete's foot is more likely to occur if you have any of the following risk factors:

Fungal growth is most prolific in warm, humid climates.

• Excessive perspiration can promote the formation of unsightly fungi in the skin and hair of the foot.

Moisture might become trapped in your feet if you wear tight, non-breathable shoes.

Public showers, locker rooms, and pool decks are prime breeding grounds for fungi, so it's best to avoid going barefoot in these locations.

- Weakened immune system: People with impaired immune systems are more susceptible.

5. To avoid getting athlete's foot, you can take these precautions:

• Wash your feet everyday and dry them completely, especially in the spaces between your toes.

• Wear shoes that let your feet breathe, such as those manufactured from natural materials.

Avoid wearing the same pair of shoes twice in a row, and switch to moisture-wicking socks to keep your feet dry.

Use shower shoes or flip-flops instead of bare feet in shared spaces like locker rooms and showers.

If you are prone to getting athlete's foot, one preventative measure is to use an antifungal powder or cream and apply it to your feet.

6. Athlete's foot can be treated using over-the-counter antifungal creams, sprays, or powders. Stronger antifungal drugs may be prescribed by a medical practitioner in more severe situations or after over-the-counter treatments have failed.

You should see a doctor if you have any reason to suspect you have athlete's foot or if your symptoms are very severe or persistent.

Hygiene and Precaution

To avoid getting sick, especially from fungal infections like athlete's foot, it's important to take precautions and maintain excellent hygiene. Some suggestions for staying healthy and clean:

1. Preserve the Health of Your Feet: Wash your feet everyday with soap and warm water. It's important to scrub in between your toes.

Fungi flourish in damp areas, so after washing your feet, be sure to dry them thoroughly, including in the spaces between your toes.

2.Put on Adequate Shoes:

• Shoes made of leather or canvas are better options since they allow air to circulate. Air can flow through them, and they'll keep your feet dry.

• Do not wear shoes that are too snug, as this might lead to foot fungus.

Socks that wick away sweat are something to think about if you value dry feet.

3. Alternate Socks and Shoes on a Routine Basis:

• Wear different shoes on different days. Shoes need time to breathe in between wears, so rotate them.

If your feet perspire a lot, you should change your socks every day.

4. Wearing Shoes Indoors:

• Wear shower shoes or flip-flops to public showers, locker rooms, or swimming pools to prevent fungal infection on your feet.

5. Maintain Regular Pedicures:

• To avoid ingrown toenails and fungal infection, it's important to keep toenails short and trimmed straight across on a regular basis.

6. Keep your belongings to yourself:

• Towels, socks, shoes, and other objects that touch your feet should not be shared. Items tainted with fungi can facilitate their spread.

7. Apply Fungicides:

• If you tend to get foot and shoe fungal infections, you might want to try using over-the-counter antifungal powders, sprays, or creams.

8. Preserve Good Sanitation:

• Take frequent showers and scrub your whole body, especially your feet, thoroughly.

After each and every bath or shower, grab a new, clean towel.

• Keep your living and sleeping areas clean and well-ventilated to prevent the formation of fungus.

9. Control Moisture and Perspiration:

• If you have especially sweaty feet, you can use foot powders or antiperspirants to assist reduce moisture.

Socks made to wick away sweat will help keep your feet dry.

10. Living a Healthy Life:

• Keep your immune system strong with a balanced diet, regular exercise, and plenty of rest. A healthy immune system can help your body fend off infections.

11. Look for redness, itching, peeling, or cracking on your feet as well as any other indicators of infection on a regular basis. You should act quickly if you experience any of these signs.

Keep in mind that excellent cleanliness is crucial for avoiding athlete's foot and for your general health and well-being. Seek medical attention for diagnosis and treatment of athlete's foot or any other chronic foot condition.

CHAPTER TWO
Evaluation and Care

Although minor instances can sometimes be treated with OTC remedies, a healthcare provider is usually needed for diagnosis and treatment of athlete's foot. The standard procedure for diagnosis and therapy is outlined below.

Diagnosis:

• The first step in diagnosing athlete's foot is a thorough physical examination, during which the doctor will look for symptoms including redness, itching, peeling, and cracking in the skin of the affected area (often the feet).

• Potassium hydroxide (KOH) preparation is a basic laboratory test that your doctor may order in specific situations. The presence of fungal components is confirmed by combining a scrape of skin from the afflicted area with KOH and then examining it under a microscope.

Treatment:

• The choice of treatment depends on the severity of the infection. While over-the-counter (OTC) remedies are usually sufficient for mild illnesses, prescription drugs may be necessary for more severe or chronic diseases:

1. Apply an antifungal cream or ointment to the affected region as instructed on the label. These may be found in most drugstores. Clotrimazole, miconazole, terbinafine, and tolnaftate are all examples of commonly used active compounds.

• Antifungal powders provide the added benefit of keeping your feet dry; they may also contain the same active ingredients found in ointments and creams.

2. Medication Requiring a Prescription

• Oral Antifungal drugs: In cases of severe or resistant infections, a healthcare provider may give oral antifungal drugs, such as fluconazole, itraconazole, or terbinafine. These drugs are usually taken for a few weeks at a time.

• If over-the-counter options aren't doing the trick, your doctor may recommend stronger topical antifungal drugs.

3. Aid at Home:

• Take the medication exactly as directed by your doctor or the package insert.

• Wash and dry your feet regularly.

• Put on shoes that let air in and socks that wick away sweat.

Towels, socks, and shoes should not be shared.

If your symptoms improve before your treatment is over, don't stop taking your medication.

4. If you have a serious infection, if your condition does not improve with treatment, or if it worsens, it is crucial that you schedule a follow-up appointment with your doctor. They may need to change your treatment strategy or rule out other possible skin disorders.

5. Following effective treatment for athlete's foot, it is important to maintain proper foot care and take other preventative steps to avoid re-infection.

Consult a doctor for a diagnosis and treatment plan if you think you have athlete's foot or if your symptoms are severe. The sooner the infection is treated, the less likely it will spread or become persistent.

Handling Difficulties

Athlete's foot is a frequent and mild ailment that responds well to therapy and good hygiene. However, complications and worsening of the infection are always possible possibilities. Here's how to treat athlete's foot in its most severe forms:

1. Scratching can spread bacteria from your nails or skin to the wound, resulting in a secondary bacterial infection. To control:

Remember to clean and trim your nails regularly.

• Try not to scratch the sore.

A doctor may recommend antibiotics if a bacterial illness develops.

2. Chronic or recurring Infections: Some persons are more prone to recurring or chronic athlete's foot. If that's the case, think about it like this:

• Discuss the matter with a healthcare physician to rule out any underlying medical disorders that may lead to repeated infections.

• Your doctor may advise you to take preventative steps over the long term, like using antifungal powders or lotions on a regular basis, or even taking oral antifungal medicine.

Recurrence can be avoided with consistent attention to foot care and other preventative measures.

3. Athlete's foot can become more difficult to cure if it spreads to the toenails (a condition known as tinea unguium). Tinea unguium describes this condition. To control:

It may take a lengthier course of oral antifungal drugs, therefore it's important to get a good diagnosis and treatment from a medical professional.

Maintain regular nail trimming and washing of the affected toes.

4. Rarely, people can have an adverse reaction to the active components in antifungal creams and other topical treatments. Stop using the antifungal treatment and see a doctor if you develop redness, swelling, or increased itching.

5. If you have diabetes or an impaired immune system, you should take athlete's foot very seriously because of the consequences it can cause. Seek advice from your doctor on how to treat the infection and lessen the likelihood of problems.

6. If you have tried over-the-counter remedies for athlete's foot but the illness persists or worsens, you should contact a doctor as soon as possible. A professional medical diagnosis allows for effective therapy, which may involve heavier prescription drugs.

Keep in mind that the key to avoiding problems is prompt diagnosis and treatment. Consult a medical professional for personalized advice and treatment options if you have questions or concerns regarding athlete's foot. In addition, preventative actions and basic foot hygiene can greatly lessen the likelihood of problems and recurrence.

CHAPTER THREE
The Athlete's Foot and Beyond

While athlete's foot is a common fungal infection that mostly affects the feet, there are other fungal infections and skin disorders that can affect various sections of the body. Fungal infections and skin disorders are not limited to athlete's foot; here are other examples:

1. Ringworm (Tinea Corporis): Ringworm is a fungal infection that can affect the skin on many regions of the body, including the arms, legs, face, and trunk. It frequently appears as a circular or ring-shaped rash and can be irritating. Antifungal creams or pills are commonly used for treatment.

2. Tinea cruris, more often known as "jock itch," is a fungal infection that primarily manifests itself in the groin, inner thighs, and buttocks. A rash, itching, and redness may result. Jock itch is typically treated with antifungal treatments.

3. Tinea versicolor is a fungal infection that manifests as blotchy discoloration of the skin, most frequently on the upper body. Patches of white, pink, or brown skin may develop. Tinea versicolor can be treated with antifungal lotions, shampoos, or pills.

4. Oral thrush, also known as thrush, is a yeast infection of the mouth. Vaginal yeast infections, also known as thrush, are an infection of the genital area. Yeast overgrowth is the root cause of these illnesses, hence antifungal drugs are the usual course of treatment.

5. Thickened, discolored, and brittle nails are symptoms of onychomycosis, a fungal infection of the nails. Antifungal creams or pills may be used in treatment.

6. Candidiasis is a fungal infection caused by the fungus Candida, which can manifest itself in a number of ways including on the skin, the nails, and the mucous membranes. Diaper rash, oral thrush, and cutaneous candidiasis are all examples of this category of skin infections. The infection's location and intensity are key factors in determining treatment.

7. Pityriasis Rosea is a skin ailment characterized by the appearance of many, progressively smaller, pink, scaly patches anywhere on the body, most frequently on the chest, back, or belly. A virus or fungus infection is probably to blame. Pityriasis rosea usually clears up on its own, however it can be treated by reducing irritation.

8. Itchy, irritated skin is a hallmark of eczema, also known as dermatitis. Although it's not a fungal infection, it can lead to fungal infections if the skin barrier is impaired. Topical corticosteroids, moisturizing, and avoiding irritants are all part of the management process.

9. Psoriasis is an ongoing skin disorder that causes red, scaly spots all over the body. While psoriasis itself is not contagious, it can be made worse by bacterial or fungal infections. Light therapy, oral medicines, and topical lotions are all potential treatments.

Consult a medical professional for a correct diagnosis and treatment plan if you think you have a fungal infection or skin disease. Location, severity, and etiology all have a role in how these disorders are treated.

Conclusion

The skin on the feet is often the first to be affected by athlete's foot, a fungal infection. Symptoms include dry, flaky skin that typically appears between the toes and on the soles of the feet, as well as itching, redness, peeling, and cracking. Good hygiene measures, such as keeping feet clean and dry, using breathable footwear, and avoiding shared personal things, are useful in preventing and treating athlete's foot.

It is crucial to see a doctor if you have any reason to suspect you have athlete's foot or if your symptoms persist or worsen. Mild instances may respond well to over-the-counter antifungal treatments, whereas chronic or severe infections may require prescription drugs.

The possibility of subsequent bacterial infections or the infection spreading to the toenails is another issue that must be considered. The key to avoiding these consequences is an early diagnosis and subsequent treatment.

There are several types of fungal infections and skin diseases beyond athlete's foot. In order to get an appropriate diagnosis and individualized treatment plan for these disorders, it is vital to see a healthcare specialist.

The best way to avoid getting a fungal infection or developing a skin problem is to practice excellent hygiene and take preventative measures. Despite their annoying nature, most of these illnesses respond well to therapy and care.

THE END